STRONG LIKE WATER GUIDED JOURNEY

T0017002

STRONG

A Compassionate Path to

LIKE

True Flourishing

WATER

GUIDED JOURNEY

AUNDI KOLBER MA LPC

AUTHOR OF *TRY SOFTER*

TYNDALE
REFRESH

Think Well. Live Well. Be Well.

Visit Tyndale online at tyndale.com.

Tyndale, Tyndale's quill logo, *Tyndale Refresh*, and the Tyndale Refresh logo are registered trademarks of Tyndale House Ministries. Tyndale Refresh is a nonfiction imprint of Tyndale House Publishers, Carol Stream, Illinois.

Strong like Water Guided Journey: A Compassionate Path to True Flourishing

Copyright © 2024 by Andrea M. Kolber. All rights reserved.

Cover photograph of painting copyright © Tracie Cheng. All rights reserved.

Author photograph copyright © 2022 by Nettie Marie Photography. All rights reserved.

Interior outline of person standing copyright © Valenty/Adobe Stock. All rights reserved.

Designed by Eva M. Winters

Published in association with Don Gates of the literary agency The Gates Group; www.the-gates-group.com.

Scripture quotations are taken from the Holy Bible, *New International Version*,® *NIV.*® Copyright © 1973, 1978, 1984, 2011 by Biblica, Inc.® Used by permission. All rights reserved worldwide.

For information about special discounts for bulk purchases, please contact Tyndale House Publishers at csresponse@tyndale.com, or call 1-855-277-9400.

The URLs in this book were verified prior to publication. The publisher is not responsible for content in the links, links that have expired, or websites that have changed ownership after that time.

The case examples in this book are fictional composites based on the author's professional interactions with hundreds of clients over the years. All names are invented, and any resemblance between these fictional characters and real people is coincidental.

ISBN 978-1-4964-5475-1

Printed in China

30	29	28	27	26	25	24
7	6	5	4	3	2	1

CONTENTS

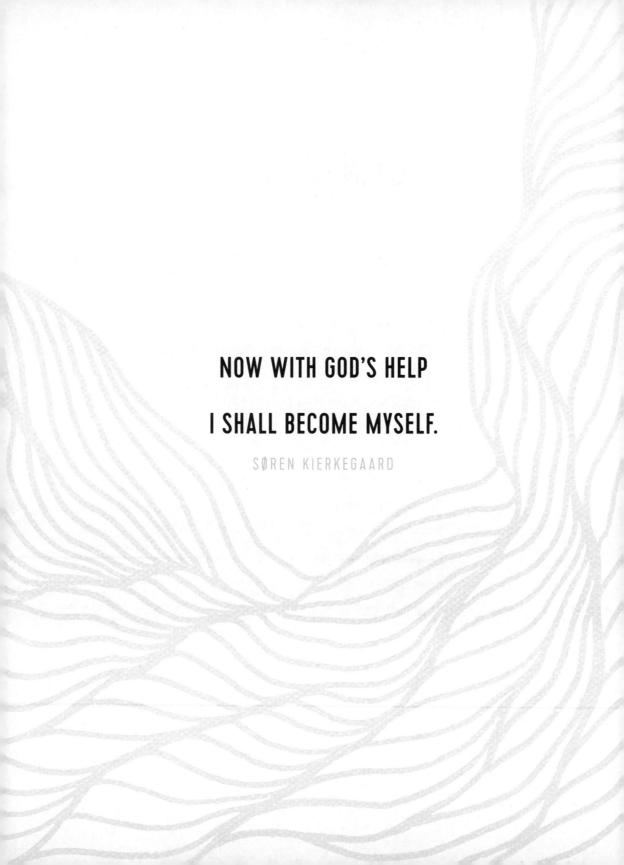

NOW WITH GOD'S HELP

I SHALL BECOME MYSELF.

SØREN KIERKEGAARD

INTRODUCTION

THE COLORADO SKY IS CLEAR; the moon shines with a pale white light even as the sun rises and begins to make her debut across the Front Range. Silently, I hand my mom her coffee, turn my keys in the ignition, and begin to drive out of our neighborhood toward the airport. My mom has been visiting for a few weeks, and now it's time for her to return home to the Pacific Northwest. We drive in easy silence for a few minutes, sipping coffee and enjoying the view.

We've come a long way, my mom and I. Much of my own story is intertwined with hers. I grew up knowing my mom loved me, but because of abuse in her marriage as well as her own history of trauma and alcoholism, she often couldn't be the mom I needed. She couldn't always protect me from my dad. Our entire family had to walk on eggshells around his psychological abuse, explosive anger, and violent punishments. As a result of my dad's rage and my mom's distance, my earliest identity was mainly formed around a sense of constant threat. I had to be stronger than a little one should ever have to be; I felt a burden to "keep it all together" so as not to cause more pain. Putting on my game face, I ventured into the world alone (or so I felt). If no one was going to show up for me, I'd find ways to survive anyway. I'd perform, tie myself in pretzels to keep others happy, and—somehow—find a way to keep going.

Yet in these last decades a precious alchemy has happened. It's not been without deep (and often painful) work—for both my mom and me. But our relationship has softened. We have witnessed and experienced what the psalmist called "the goodness of the LORD in the land of the living" (Psalm 27:13). Through experiences of support, safety, therapy, education, and the nearness of God, my life is on a different trajectory than I have any business being on.

And so here we drive, my mom and I.

After we reminisce about her visit, our conversation begins to turn toward more weighty matters. It almost seems that as we get closer to the airport, we move closer to the truth of who we are. We talk about things like healing, questions, and even doubts. We talk about how things could have been different. We talk about anger. We talk about grief. We talk about the ways we don't understand the mystery of God but know He is with us.

"Aundi, honey," she says—her voice cracking—"you're more tenacious now than you ever were as a young basketball player." She laughs to herself. "And that's saying something. Because I remember the way you used to play."

It's true. The strength that carried me through life was never more evident than when I was on the court. I turn the car into the drop-off lane—our time together is almost done. My mom's voice grows quiet. "But you're more gentle too," she whispers. "I love seeing who you've become."

My hands grip the steering wheel and tears start to stream down my face. It's deeply validating to hear my mom say these words to me; I sense that she is perceiving me in a way she wasn't able to in my childhood. She is seeing all of me—more than just my survival strength—and calling it good.

My mom has said what I have learned to be true: There is a different way for me to be strong.

AN INVITATION: A FLEXIBLE AND EXPANSIVE GUIDE

It has taken me years to learn that I can be both soft and strong; that in fact, my strength sustains my softness, and my softness is a resource to my strength. That like the ocean I grew up next to, we each have so much more depth than is visible on the surface; God designed each of us like an entire universe.

And how about you, dear one? Do you know what it's like to feel afraid of your own story or your own life? Are you exhausted trying to live from the kind of strength that's been required of you to keep going—but wonder what other choice you have?

I get it.

Sometimes I wish I didn't. There have been times in my own journey and my work with clients when grief has felt like a deep cavern. And yet, I'd like to tell you one of the things that my dear friend Tasha Jun once wrote as we honor our strong-like-water work. She said this: "Lament is a womb for hope."[1]

Reader, it is my deep prayer that our work in the pages ahead will feel more like a "womb" than a tomb. That as we dive deeper into this expansive way to be in the world, you will begin to internalize the idea that strength doesn't have to look just one way—and it doesn't have to cost you yourself. It's so much bigger and more inclusive than you can imagine. And as you begin to embody this idea, I pray you can utilize some of the resources provided to honor your grief, your questions, and your fears—even as you open up to possibilities of healing.

I wish I could tell you this work is going to be easy and fast. Don't we all, on some level, want to figure out how we can heal *right now*? It is extremely tempting and very human of us to want immediate change.

And yet, that's just not how this work *works*. This is a journey of a lifetime, and we know that we may never see full healing on this side of heaven.

But I will say this: Just because the work is difficult, it doesn't mean there won't be moments of ease in your journey. In fact, every single time you begin to engage your story—body, mind, and spirit—from a lens of safety and compassion, you're *already* healing. Just the fact that you are here with a heart beating in your chest, curious about how to become more of who God made you to be, is a beautiful symbol of the goodness in you and a sign of the growth to come.

I've done my best to structure the *Strong like Water Guided Journey* in the most accessible, gentle, and effective way possible to accommodate both growth and compassion. Though it's good and necessary for us to stretch ourselves at times, for many trauma survivors, hearing that they need to get even *more* uncomfortable in order to grow, heal, or change can be quite overwhelming. This is incredibly valid, of course. You may have spent your whole life in survival mode, completely outside your comfort zone. Because this is true, I do all I can to work from what is known as a trauma-informed lens. With almost every practice, I will prompt you to check in with yourself to make sure your nervous system isn't flooded or disconnected to prevent any harm as we go along. Similarly, I will always try to empower you with choices, reminding you that you can do any and all of the practices ahead at your own pace and in the ways that best serve you; or you can choose not to do them at all. If you'd like to skip sections to come back to later or complete some content partially, you may absolutely do so. In many ways, the internal attunement you practice in doing that is just as much of your strong-like-water work as anything else.

Within the guided journey, I have separated the work into five distinct sections that will enhance various topics from *Strong like Water*.[2] In order to help enrich what you've already learned from the book, what we discuss in these sections will connect, build on, or expand on the principles in a deeper, more reflective way.

Here's a closer look at what you might expect as we continue:

Holding Space for Our Stories

One of the most beautiful concepts I've come to learn both professionally and personally is that stories change and move us. Not only that, but each of us carries our own story of lived experience in our body. At the beginning of each section, you'll find a short personal reflection to help you continue processing concepts learned in the corresponding *Strong like Water* chapters. You can also find a free, short video introduction for these ideas on my website: aundikolber.com/slwvideos. (Use the password stronglikewater.)

Body-Centered Exercise

The work we do in *Strong like Water* is not for the faint of heart. It can be hard and painful, deep soul work that requires compassion and gentleness. You learned in *Strong like Water* how to check in with yourself and your body, and while I invite you to do this throughout the guided journey, each session will also allow space to explicitly focus on your body. These practices are an extension of what you'll have learned in the corresponding chapters of *Strong like Water* and are meant to help you anchor the content we're working through in your whole self. With that said, safety is key: You'll notice that I often provide cues to make sure you're accessing body work in a way and at a tempo that feels doable to you. Please know that regardless of the extent to which you engage in these practices, just by honoring the pace of your body and your innate need for safety, you are already beginning the work of healing.

Invitation to Reflect and Discuss

While much of the strong-like-water work will be individual, God wired our bodies for interpersonal connection and co-regulation. If you want to do this work in an authentic and supportive group environment, you can adapt and facilitate accordingly. The questions are meant to spark introspection and reflection—as well as conversation and sharing to the extent that you feel comfortable. Because this is such vulnerable and personal work, I've included a short resource, "Guidance for Group Leaders," that highlights core components of trauma-informed communication, which you'll find in the back of this book. Especially in groups, creating and maintaining safety are of utmost importance. Be intentional about cultivating a space of trust—and give each other permission to participate and interact with the material *as you personally choose to*. You are the best judge of how much of your story and your experience feels helpful to disclose. My hope is that realizing you are not alone on this journey of living strong like water will be a balm of encouragement to your soul.

Invitation to Journal

Much of the deep work of compassionate resourcing happens squarely within your mind, body, and psyche, and this journaling section is one way to continue to attune to your own story. Many of the prompts I've written are similar to questions and activities I would delve into with you if we were sitting in my therapy office. My hope is that as you engage with these questions, they will provide a springboard that allows you to gently hold and honor the complexities of your personhood.

Invitation to Create

Have you ever noticed that some experiences are hard to describe with words? Or have you ever felt like words aren't enough? We all experience this from time to time, but it can be especially true when parts of our stories have been distressing or traumatic. This is why I want to invite you to use art to gently tap into your right brain, which researchers note is connected to imagery, symbolism, emotion, and sensation.[3] Even when parts of your story aren't distressing, finding ways to access the right brain can be helpful as you move toward integration and wholeness—for it is from a place of deeper integration that you can continue to resource and pay compassionate attention to the wounds that are still aching.

In this "Invitation to Create" section, feel free to adapt the prompts so they best empower you as you honor your story. And as a sidenote, don't let your perceived lack of artistic skill keep you from trying these. Many of us wouldn't consider ourselves artists, and that's okay! As with all our work, the process of creating is as important as what we've created, no matter how it turns out.

Reader, in a culture that often misunderstands the courage required to truly heal, I believe you are wildly brave for engaging in this strong-like-water work. I'm not sure how you're arriving at these pages: whether anxious and frayed or bruised and weary—or perhaps somewhere in between. But I am so glad you're here. I believe you matter; the intricacies of your life and personhood matter. They matter not only to me as a fellow image bearer, but to our world and to the God who formed you. May I offer an even more audacious hope: I pray you come to know that it's possible—truly possible—to heal and live into a more expansive strength, even if you start with only a glimpse of that strength. I pray that in the work ahead, you will experience a sense of alignment with the person you were created to be and the presence of the Spirit of God, who loves you profoundly.

ONE WAVE AT A TIME

MORGAN HARPER NIC•HOLS

COMPASSION MEANS

FULL IMMERSION IN THE CONDITION

OF BEING HUMAN.

HENRI J. M. NOUWEN, *SHOW ME THE WAY*

EMBODIED PAIN REQUIRES EMBODIED HEALING

A Deeper Dive into Chapters 1 and 2 of *Strong like Water*

"WOW, CHARLOTTE, UM, WHAT A STORY," Izzy said distractedly. "You've been so strong pushing through this." As she talked, Izzy riffled through her wallet and tried to get the server's attention, signaling that lunch was over.

Charlotte was stunned by Izzy's nonchalance; she had just shared about the intense betrayal she'd experienced at the hands of a coworker to whom she'd once felt close. This experience had upended Charlotte's entire life, forcing her to resign from her job and lose most of her support network. Even more, it had rattled her faith. She felt alone, confused, and disoriented by the loss of this friendship. For Charlotte, telling this story was a major deal, a vulnerable sharing of her wounded heart. Just the emotional exhaustion from talking about her experience required courage that Charlotte hadn't been sure she possessed. Though Izzy was saying the right words of validation, somehow they rang hollow.

Charlotte's hands felt clammy as she took the last bite of her meal. Suddenly she felt a rush of shame, the heat filling her face. Had Izzy even wanted to hear her story? Why had sharing this tender part with her made Charlotte feel *worse*, not better, like she'd thought it would? Why did she feel even more alone? An intense sensation of heaviness settled in her; she just wanted to leave the restaurant immediately and hide.

Instead, she did what she always did. She pasted on a smile, suppressing the millions of emotions actually coming up. Then—and Charlotte felt especially angry at herself for this—*she* apologized to Izzy for being such a "high-maintenance friend" who was so "needy."

Izzy smiled back and said, "Well, yes—sometimes you are."

In the moment, Charlotte couldn't seem to avoid falling right back into her old habits of overaccommodating and overfunctioning at the expense of her own well-being. Charlotte felt deeply conflicted by her actions, and yet she didn't know what else to do.

Later that night, Charlotte tried to reflect on the missed connection at lunch. She knew Izzy meant well, and she did try to be supportive. Charlotte appreciated that. But even so, she felt *missed*. Like Izzy hadn't truly seen her. Like Izzy hadn't been there for her, not really. Like at the end of the day, Charlotte had to get through this trial on her own.

This wasn't a new feeling for Charlotte, and it had started way before her friendship with Izzy. Charlotte was the oldest of three kids in a family that valued responsibility and hard work. She was used to needing to figure things out on her own. As Charlotte was growing up, her parents had come down brutally on her if she spoke up or asked for more support because they wanted her to be prepared for "the hard world out there." She loved her parents, but they often micromanaged her schoolwork and extracurriculars to make sure she was succeeding. Through all the stress, Charlotte was expected to maintain a positive attitude no matter how much she was hurting or what she faced. Even when tragedy struck and she lost her dearest friend in a car accident when she was only in middle school, Charlotte knew there wasn't any real space for her to grieve. Even though her parents told her they supported her and it was okay to cry, their actions told a different story.

It seemed to be like that with everyone Charlotte loved: They appeared to be there for her, but after the lights went out and she was alone, she often felt isolated and unsupported, like she was the only one in the universe.

Charlotte was so tired of always being strong—at least the kind of strong she thought people like Izzy and her parents wanted from her. Recently, Charlotte had been trying to be more aware of this exhaustion, to heal from how these relationships made her feel. However, her efforts—wellness retreats, diets, prayer hacks, cleanses, and forms of therapy focused on changing her thoughts—worked only temporarily, and when she didn't notice lasting change, ultimately she felt more shame.

There had to be more to life than this. A fuller, more connected way of living. But how would she ever find it?

Many of us, like Charlotte, have learned that strength seems to always involve pushing down what we truly need and pushing ourselves beyond our limits so that we ultimately live a life that's fractured from our true sense of self. This is operating in survival mode—or as I call it, situational strength. But please remember, this kind of strong is not bad. It serves a very distinct and necessary purpose: navigating overwhelming, disturbing, and/or life-threatening experiences. And thank goodness we have the ability to tap into this type of strength, because the fact that God designed our bodies to survive is a gift. But its purpose was *never* to sustain us permanently.

As with Charlotte, too often what begins as an adaptive strength in one situation becomes our default strength in all situations. It becomes our reflexive position as we move through life. It's as if our bodies carry the imprint of past pain into the next moment because we never fully metabolized that hurt in the first place. So we survive, yes, but we never thrive because we aren't experiencing the fullness God created us for.

What alternatives do we have? We begin by working to understand that it was never pain that made us strong in the first place. That we don't need to celebrate pain to cultivate strength. After all, our ability not only to survive but also to heal has always been a gift from our Creator—it's been within us from the start.

The reality is that, like water, our bodies and emotions are designed to flow between nervous system states and ultimately toward wholeness. Yet unfortunately, our experiences of unresolved pain and trauma impede that movement, and instead of processing through them, the pain gets stuck. Many of us have lived our lives like Charlotte, constantly slapping on a smile in the face of deep despair.

But through attuned therapy and the slow building of a few friendships committed to genuine reciprocity, Charlotte began to learn she had always been worthy of love and care. It was slow work, especially at first, but this care birthed courage in her to build her resources, set boundaries, and begin to move through the world as more herself than she had ever been.

This is possible for you, too, my friend. My conceptualization of the flow of strength (see page 5) helps us imagine the practicalities of how our bodies wisely adapt and integrate as we begin to gain the compassionate resources we need and embody strength like water. Each of the three types of strength serves a purpose and gives us vital information about our needs, process, and experience:

Situational strength: Our bodies operate from a stress/trauma response to navigate or neutralize difficulty. We are reacting from a neurobiological level rather than conscious choice, and in the absence of enough safety after the difficulties occur, our experiences may remain fragmented in our bodies and minds.

Transitional strength: As we experience cues of safety, we have the capacity to attend to the wounded and traumatized parts of ourselves, offering them resources and support. We learn to hold dichotomies, understanding we may have pain but that it is not our identity. Similarly, we learn to hold both goodness and sorrow; joy and suffering. As a result, we begin to have a choice in how we engage our stories, bodies, and strength.

Integrated strength: Through care and support, our bodies are able to digest the intensity we have felt and the pain that has plagued us. We gain the capacity to learn from and reflect on our experiences, and the wounded parts of ourselves experience various levels of repair. Increasing levels of internal safety give us the capabilities to extend love, hope, and safety to ourselves and others.

THE FLOW OF STRENGTH

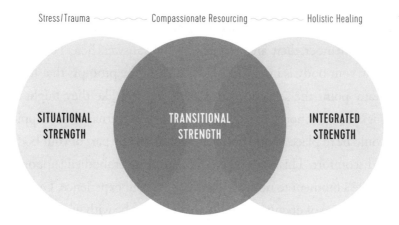

Stress/Trauma ～～～ Compassionate Resourcing ～～～ Holistic Healing

SITUATIONAL STRENGTH

TRANSITIONAL STRENGTH

INTEGRATED STRENGTH

Though different types of strength are required in different situations, compassionate resourcing (safety and support) is the current that moves us along the flow of strength toward a more holistic and sustainable way to be in the world.

Learning to identify and flow between each, then, is the source of our most expansive strength. Our power comes not from the wounds, but the tending. Not from the trauma, but from the way it's cared for. Love is the building block for true resilience.

BODY-CENTERED EXERCISE

I'm a big advocate of compassionate resourcing, the idea of "*coming alongside and remaining responsive to* the parts of ourselves and our stories that *do not yet* feel safe" (*Strong like Water*, page 75). Psychologist Dr. Arielle Schwartz defines such resources as "anything that communicates safety to our bodies in the present."[1] For our first body-centered exercise, then, I want to remind you of several foundational resources to build safety such as grounding and containment. You'll find them on pages 95 and 96. If you've traveled with me through both *Try Softer* and *Strong like Water*, you know that these resources are where I always begin; truly, their importance cannot be overstated.

Now, as you're able, take a moment to do a body scan while reflecting on each of the types of strength. Picture a laser going over your body from the top of your head down to your toes, noticing any sensations or emotions that may come up. Remember, there are no right or wrong answers here. For now, simply notice how your body is interacting with each of the prompts that follow.

If at any point the sensations that come up feel like they might be overwhelming, you can choose to stop this activity. An alternative to stopping altogether could be to place a hand on your chest or on any part of your body where you feel discomfort. This is a way you may provide embodied support to your system. Take a moment to notice if that changes your experience. Do you notice softening? A sense of opening? A sense that you can be with what is coming up?

1. A body-centered lens in therapy reminds us that the sensations and emotions that are evoked when we reflect on a concept, memory, or event are vital information. In a way, we can consider this a means by which our body "speaks" to us even below

our cognitive stories. For this next exercise, I want to guide you through getting curious about what comes up in your own body when we reflect on the various types of strength.

Take a moment to think about the concept of situational strength: the kind of strength that may feel like your only option when you're trying to survive, no matter the cost. As you're able, consider what you're noticing in your own body as you reflect on the concept. (Notice that we're just reflecting on the concept, not necessarily the situation that put you in that state.) You may notice straining, clenching, overextending, or even feeling disconnected, trapped, contracted, heavy, or more. (As much as possible, simply observe these sensations without getting lost in them.) Where in your body do you feel these sensations? If it's helpful, mark them below.

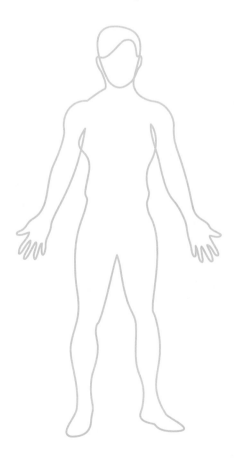

2. Now, consider what you notice in your body when you think about moving toward transitional strength: the kind of strength in which you feel at least a bit secure. You may have one foot in survival mode, but you have some resources that enable you to cope—perhaps even to move through your emotion.

   To begin this exercise, take a moment to orient yourself to the room you are in. Pay attention to what you see, hear, and smell. This is a means to come back to the present moment while still honoring what your body is telling you. Once you've allowed your senses to establish you right where you are, use a body scan to observe what you are experiencing internally as you consider transitional strength. Do you notice any shifts in sensations or emotions as you consider what resources are available to you? A lightness? A sense of being able to observe your experience rather than getting lost in it? You may even want to jot a few notes below. This interplay of being *with yourself* as you consider transitional strength is a way to begin to attend to yourself.

3. Finally, I invite you to do a body scan as you consider the concept of integrated strength: the kind of strength that comes from knowing—deep within you—that you have worked through something hard. Often there's a sense of completion, settledness, or embodied knowing of who you are and what you need in that moment. You may notice a feeling of hopefulness, peace, or clarity. And if you have rarely experienced integrated strength in your own life, that is completely okay. For now, we are simply assessing how your body is responding to the concepts. If you'd like, use the space below to write a few notes.

SOMATIC VOCABULARY

An important part of moving trauma and stress through your body is learning to tune in and describe your bodily sensations.[2] Once you do so, you can decide how to move or otherwise support your body so that the feeling doesn't remain stuck inside you.

This vocabulary list might be a good starting point for you, but I encourage you to remain curious and add your own words as you learn to attune to the sensations of your body.

· achy	· hot	· soggy
· airy	· light	· tender
· anchored	· loose	· tense
· buzzy	· lukewarm	· tight
· clear	· open	· tingly
· cold	· pointy	· trembling
· contracted	· prickly	· vibrating
· electric	· pulsing	· wobbly
· expansive	· radiating	·
· full	· rough	·
· fuzzy	· satiated	·
· grounded	· saturated	·
· hard	· small	·
· heavy	· smooth	·

INVITATION TO REFLECT AND DISCUSS

1. When you think of someone you consider strong, who comes to mind? In your view, how does this person embody strength? Now that you are familiar with the flow of strength, which type of strength does this person seem to embody most?

2. Have you ever felt like you needed to pretend you were okay when you weren't? Or similarly, have you shied away from being honest with others about how you are feeling because you fear doing so wouldn't be received well? If you can, describe that sensation—what did it feel like, emotionally and physically?

3. In *Strong like Water*, I note that "in temporary, short spurts, situational strength is extremely helpful, necessary, and even protective" (page 21). When has situational strength helped or protected you? Which of the situational strength strategies in the table on pages 26–29 of *Strong like Water* feel especially familiar to you?

4. As you feel able, consider why you've perceived that you need to be "the strong one" in the first place. Though it may not be possible or even desirable to continue to live from situational strength, in what ways do you think your body might have done so to try to protect you?

5. What do you believe God's posture toward you is when you are in pain or survival mode? Where do you think this belief stems from?

6. "Love changes us in ways that fear and danger cannot" (*Strong like Water*, page 36). What do you think that means? Has that ever been true in your own experience? In what ways does this feel connected to the verse "Perfect love drives out fear" (1 John 4:18)?

7. What do you think it might mean to honor pain? What is the difference between honoring pain and trying to fix it?

8. In *Strong like Water* (pages 50–52), we discuss the idea that there is a difference between discomfort and harm. If you feel comfortable doing so, consider whether you are able to distinguish between discomfort and harm in your own system. How do you know the difference? What cues let you know you may be moving toward harm in your own body, relationships, or experience?

INVITATION TO JOURNAL

Have you ever felt like you've had to be "the strong one"? If so, why?

How does a strong-like-water perspective challenge what you've been taught? How might that change how you're showing up to your life?

If it feels helpful, consider how often strength is viewed as a paradox in Scripture (e.g., "When I am weak, then I am strong" [2 Corinthians 12:10]; "Unless you change and become like little children, you will never enter the kingdom of heaven" [Matthew 18:3]). If doing so feels like a resource, consider how that paradoxical lens might affect your perspective on strength.

A PRAYER FOR HONORING

As you feel comfortable, find a safe space and settle into these words.
You might even put your hand on your heart and, after reading through the
prayer, close your eyes to reflect further:

*God, here in this moment, empower me to honor everything that
arises in my body, mind, and soul today; even if it means I have
to return to it at another time.*

*Creator of all things, remind me that in honoring my experiences,
You help me affirm dignity to the parts of myself that have at
times felt stripped of it.*

*God, help me know that my desire for safety and connection is
valid. In Your wisdom You designed me to need both.*

*But as I'm able, grant me the ability to open up to the possibilities
of healing and newness while staying connected to the reality of
Your love.*[3]

INVITATION TO CREATE

The concept of water is overflowing with meaning and metaphor; even the way it can change from ice to liquid to gas provides phenomenally rich images. In one way, in fact, water's mutability mirrors the way we can learn to be flexible in the stages of our strength, flowing from one form to another depending on our situation.

Of course we know that water—which makes up about 60 percent of our bodies—is vital to our very existence.[4] Though water is critical for physical life, throughout the Bible water is often used symbolically to convey our spiritual need as well. The Gospel writers point out that Jesus is the One who can truly quench our "thirst." As Jesus said, "Everyone who drinks this water will be thirsty again, but whoever drinks the water I give them will never thirst. Indeed, the water I give them will become in them a spring of water welling up to eternal life" (John 4:13-14).

At other times, water represents the struggles we have to overcome or work through:

> When you pass through the waters,
>   I will be with you;
> and when you pass through the rivers,
>   they will not sweep over you.
> When you walk through the fire,
>   you will not be burned;
>   the flames will not set you ablaze.

ISAIAH 43:2

Interestingly, as different as these metaphors are, each reveals a new truth: God is both our life-giver and the life force that sustains us even when we travel through threat. I also love that there are layers of complexity to each picture. As one of my former colleagues would say, "It's all grist for the mill." Each way of looking at water can spur us on to listen to and honor the internal landscape God designed within us, as well as the ways we are invited to partake of the "living water"—Jesus Himself.

For this first creative activity, I invite you to consider the ways that water has impacted your own life. Where have you experienced it as life-giving? Does that memory or the experience of water itself feel like a resource to you? Where, if at all, has it felt treacherous? I invite you to take a moment to sketch or paint what comes to mind as you think of these scenarios. As you do, notice what colors, shapes, or themes you are drawn to. Does any poetry, Scripture, or music come to mind as you create? What are your takeaways from what you are noticing?

The truth is, having to live from situational strength can be quite costly. That's not to say there aren't ways for us to work *with* what we're carrying, but it is important to acknowledge the weight and reality of it.

As you consider this, I invite you to take a moment and review the "Getting to Know Your Container" exercise from page 59 in *Strong like Water*. Reflect on the challenges, pain, or trauma that may be filling up your container while staying connected to your own window of tolerance (the range of arousal in which you can feel or experience something in a way that is tolerable to your body). Consider how you might express what you're carrying—not through words, but through painting or drawing. What colors appeal to you? Which shapes? Do you want to take up a little space on the page or a lot? Do you notice any relief or shift as you let the paper also hold what you're carrying?

WHAT ARE YOU CARRYING?

Examples of what might be filling your "container":

a history of unresolved trauma	a demanding job
racism	job loss
anxiety	loneliness
depression	discrimination
chronic illness	caregiving
other health issues	poverty

You may be carrying other heavy experiences, including the day-to-day stressors of life that may not feel "disturbing" on their own but that when paired with everything else might lead you to rely on situational strength.

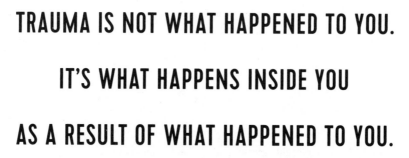

TRAUMA IS NOT WHAT HAPPENED TO YOU.

IT'S WHAT HAPPENS INSIDE YOU

AS A RESULT OF WHAT HAPPENED TO YOU.

DR. GABOR MATÉ

TENDING THE ACHE FOR COMPASSIONATE WITH-NESS

A Deeper Dive into Chapters 3 and 4 of *Strong like Water*

DURING THE SEVENTEEN YEARS I have worked as a therapist, our understanding of trauma—and how to treat it—has evolved significantly, particularly in the last decade. Unfortunately, a lack of knowledge can sometimes lead to further confusion and harm in the therapy room, an environment that is supposed to be safe and secure.

In my early twenties, I met with a therapist as I tried to do my own therapeutic "work," even as I trained for this profession. I continually felt off as I tried to reconcile what I was learning with what I was experiencing. It just didn't match; no matter how much I knew the "right" thing to do or think, it didn't change how I felt in my body—which often was anxious, alone, and unsafe. One afternoon as I sat in my then-therapist's office, I hit a breaking point. It was a warm summer Colorado day, and a fan whirred overhead. I took a deep breath and began to share an awful story involving my father. Though we had been estranged for several years, my dad continually sent me abusive letters and voice mails; he falsely accused me of actions, threatening me and trying to shame me into contacting him.

Even though I never answered, I couldn't deny how it was affecting me: I stopped checking the mail because the dread left me breathless. I panicked when my phone rang so I avoided answering at all. I was hypervigilant and afraid, ruminating on worst-case scenarios and extreme outcomes. As a kid, I'd constantly felt like I was in trouble and was afraid of his volatile mood and explosive anger—I walked on eggshells, always. I had hoped that becoming an adult would cause me to feel more empowered around these issues, but so far, it hadn't worked.

As I began to share with my therapist the details of the most recent letter, I found myself at a loss for words—my thoughts inarticulate and fragmented. My body began to tremble; I shook so severely that my teeth started to chatter. I looked down at my hands, which I simply couldn't keep still. Even though it was in the nineties outside, I was freezing. What was happening to me? Why couldn't I just relay a simple incident?

I tried to continue telling my story, but a part of me grew more and more anxious, even as I felt outside myself at the same time. Did my therapist notice what was happening and how my body was reacting as I spoke? What was the significance of my body's response—or was I simply making up this reaction in my head? As I searched my therapist's face, it remained blank. Seemingly unaware of what I was experiencing, he continued to give me well-meaning theoretical feedback, offering suggestions about how to reframe my outlook on the situation.

Whatever advice he was giving—it didn't land. The spirit was willing, but my body, she was gone, completely outside of (what I now understand as) my window of tolerance. Even though I was simply relaying a story, its connection to my dad put my body into a profound state of threat. And she was trying to save me.

After the appointment, I still shook, though I had settled a little. By the time I got home, I felt even more hopeless and alone than when I'd started the session. Was this how things would be for me? Was I doing therapy wrong? Would anyone truly *see* me? Would I ever be truly safe?

Reader, I share that story with you for a few reasons. First, if you've had experiences of trying to heal or grow that have left you feeling more wounded, alone, or in anguish, I hear you. You are not the only one. You are not bad and there is nothing to be ashamed of. We each deserve to be witnessed and honored with dignity, especially in our deepest pain. And if that hasn't been your experience, I am so sorry you've sustained that.

But perhaps equally important, I share this story to show you just what powerful communicators our bodies are. Had I or my therapist known what was happening in my body, I would have understood that you can't logic yourself out of a trauma response. I didn't need information, I needed presence. I needed compassionate with-ness. I needed to experience safety to help my body navigate the threat. The reality is, *none of us* can bypass our bodies. Understanding that our bodies are wired and designed to react to safety or threat is an important part of our strong-like-water work.

In my own story, my therapist didn't have the lens to recognize that a present-day issue with my dad was disturbing in the present—but also activating a visceral trauma response from decades of past trauma. And unfortunately, my therapist simply didn't have the understanding or training to adequately guide me to safety.

Now as a trauma therapist myself, I understand the truth: My body had gone into a freeze response and was trying to "shake its way out."[1] Similar to the way that animals in the wild have to discharge energy after they experience a life-or-death moment, so, too, do we humans. For decades, I'd lived with an abusive parent, which led to the same life-or-death feeling in my body. That's why, even though I was an adult who lived several states away from my father, I still shook.

WE EACH DESERVE TO

BE WITNESSED AND

HONORED WITH DIGNITY,

ESPECIALLY IN

OUR DEEPEST PAIN.

Here is what I've learned in the years since: There is hope. There are many ways we can learn to find safety again after we have known great harm. We can harness the language of our bodies to understand what we need—and then participate with God, others, and ourselves in offering it to our wounds. Back then, I thought suppressing my body's information was necessary for me to be strong. But I now know that there are many ways to work with my body in moving through pain rather than staying stuck in it. If it feels helpful, take a moment to review the felt safety diagram below and consider where you have opportunities to continue building safety (or savor where you already have).

WORKING TO BUILD EXPERIENCES OF FELT SAFETY

Our experience of felt safety, according to therapist Deb Dana, is the result of everything that occurs inside us, outside us, and between us. It's important to remember that our experience of safety is perceived and not necessarily literal. This is why, even when the world is tumultuous or hard, it's possible for us to work toward felt safety with ourselves and others.

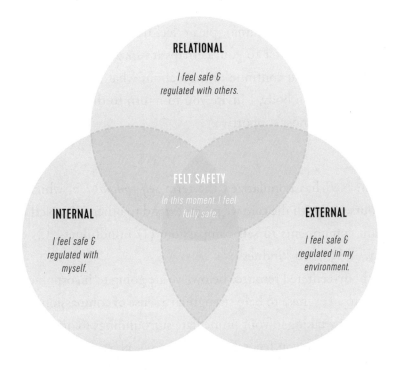

RELATIONAL

*I feel safe &
regulated with others.*

FELT SAFETY

*In this moment, I feel
fully safe.*

INTERNAL

*I feel safe &
regulated with
myself.*

EXTERNAL

*I feel safe &
regulated in my
environment.*

BODY-CENTERED EXERCISE

The concept of safety is emphasized throughout *Strong like Water*. Take a moment and consider the word *safe* for yourself. As you do, I invite you to bring your awareness to your body. What do you notice in your body? Do you tense up? What is the quality of your breath? Do you notice a softening anywhere in your body? How is your posture? Do you sense an openness in your chest? Please remember there are no right or wrong answers to this question. If the word *safety* doesn't feel like a resource to you, please skip to the space immediately below. However, if the word feels like a resource, you may consider repeating one of the following affirmations:

I deserve to feel safe.
In this moment I am safe.

If the word *safe* or *safety* is difficult for you (which it is for some, especially people with a history of trauma), please feel free to replace that word with something that feels better to you. Perhaps it's *steady, settled, regulated, connected,* or *calm.* As you continue to learn about what a sense of equilibrium feels like in your own body, I invite you to return to this exercise, using the language that feels most supportive.

Dr. Kristin Neff has popularized the term *self-compassion,* which involves treating ourselves with the care we might extend to others. Dr. Neff identifies three main components to self-compassion: (1) mindfulness, (2) common humanity, and (3) self-kindness.[2]

In the body-centered resource below, we are going to incorporate all three elements into an exercise to help strengthen a sense of compassion in our own bodies. Begin by taking in your immediate surroundings to orient yourself in your space to ensure you feel safe (mindfulness). Next, imagine someone in your life whom you care about making one of these comments about themselves (common humanity):

My pain doesn't matter.
I'm not allowed to feel.
I'm selfish to feel.
I'm too much if I feel.
I'm alone in my pain.

As you take in these phrases and see in your mind's eye this person who is dear to you, what do you notice in your own body? What sensations? Emotions? Do you have a sense of wanting to help them? To tell them something different? As you are able, I invite you to first visualize caring for the person who is feeling that way. What might you say to them? What might you do?

Finally, can you also visualize a version of yourself sitting next to the person who is hurting? Is it possible to lend some of the compassion you feel for that person toward *yourself* too (self-kindness)? Might you be able to send a little of the softness or care you feel in the direction of your own pain? As you do this, notice how your body is responding. Is it easy or difficult to offer yourself that kindness? If it's difficult, you may wish to place a hand on your heart, then see if you can take a moment to get curious about sharing even a fraction of the compassion you're feeling for the other person and extending it toward yourself. In this way, you continue to learn to love your neighbor, but also yourself. (As always, you can only go at the pace your body will allow, so if self-compassion isn't yet accessible for you, you may wish simply to observe that for now.)

INVITATION TO REFLECT AND DISCUSS

1. Why do you think vulnerability, gentleness, or expressions of emotion are often viewed as weaknesses in our culture? Do you think it's possible to access true safety without connecting to those qualities?

2. In the opening essay for this session, I discuss how much intensity I was experiencing in my body—but also my sense that I wasn't being seen or understood by my therapist. Have you ever felt as if what you were experiencing internally was not honored by those around you? If you feel comfortable sharing, explain how this affected you.

3. In *Strong like Water*, I tell the story of Georgia, an outwardly successful woman who constantly felt anxiety and dread. As much as she longed to take in the goodness and love of those around her, she struggled to do so (pages 69–76). Have you, like Georgia, tried to make a change or implement something new, only to discover that it felt too hard? What are some ways you could "start small" to practice building safety in that area of your life?

4. Deb Dana has written that trauma requires us to develop "patterns of protection" instead of "patterns of connection."[3] This means that rather than prioritizing safety that connects us (relational vulnerability, compassionate with-ness, etc.), we prioritize safety that protects us (defense mechanisms, isolation, etc.). What do you think is the difference between a type of safety that is rooted in protection and safety that is rooted in connection (see *Strong like Water*, pages 69–74)? Where in your own life may you be enacting a pattern of protection over one of connection?

5. Is there an attachment style that you lean toward? On pages 94–100 of *Strong like Water*, I discuss resources for different attachment styles. Which one or two strategies resonate with you most? Why?

6. "God *with* us is the clearest invitation to secure attachment we could ever hope for" (*Strong like Water*, page 103). What do you think this means? How do you think experiencing attachment trauma in relationships or from spiritual figures affects our ability to experience God *with* us?

7. If you feel comfortable sharing, name a place or time in your life in which you experienced a tangible sense of God with you. If you haven't had that experience personally, have you encountered someone else's story, a piece of art, a song, or a part of Scripture that evokes that sense of God's with-ness to you? If you feel comfortable sharing, describe that encounter.

INVITATION TO JOURNAL

On pages 85–87 of *Strong like Water*, I reflect on my experience with my husband, Brendan, during one of the most painful moments of my life—my final visit to my childhood home. In that moment, his presence and solidarity gave me compassionate with-ness. Take a moment to reflect on your own life. Can you describe a time when you've experienced compassionate with-ness, whether from another person, God, nature, a pet, etc.?

Compassionate with-ness can initiate a move toward transitional strength in our healing journey. As you reflect on your experience, I invite you to consider whether those moments have inspired and empowered you to treat yourself differently in moments of pain (i.e., to become your own compassionate witness to the challenges you've endured).

Finally, you might reflect on whether both types of experiences (receiving compassionate with-ness and/or learning to be your own compassionate witness) have influenced how you participate with God in your own healing journey.

WE CAN HARNESS THE LANGUAGE OF
OUR BODIES TO UNDERSTAND WHAT
WE NEED—AND THEN PARTICIPATE
WITH GOD, OTHERS, AND OURSELVES IN
OFFERING IT TO OUR WOUNDS.

INVITATION TO CREATE

For this activity, you will need crayons, pens, watercolors, or anything that helps you create.[4] Now consider again the word *safe* (or you may choose a different word if you did so in the body-centered exercise).

Take a moment and draw/paint/create a picture or representation of safety. Your creation may be literal or symbolic—whatever feels helpful to you. Additionally, you may consider whether different parts of you need different kinds of safety. For example, you may have different ages of yourself who connect with different representations of what *safe* means. Please feel free to interpret this creative prompt in the way that feels most supportive to you.

If it feels like a resource to you, I also invite you to list different experiences you've had that might be included in the relational safety, internal safety, and external safety circles in the diagram on page 39. By doing this, you are building touch points to come back to when you may be struggling to build safety in a current moment.

RELATIONAL

INTERNAL

EXTERNAL

LIFE TAUGHT YOU HOW TO FIGHT.

MAY LOVE TEACH YOU HOW TO LIVE.

DR. THEMA BRYANT

THE WISDOM OF GOODNESS

A Deeper Dive into Chapters 5 and 6 of *Strong like Water*

"AUNDI, ALL MY LIFE I've ached for affirmation from the people who don't really want me," Sharee told me as we began our session.

I settled into my seat, listening intently. I realized that a statement like this was hugely significant. I hadn't worked with Sharee for long, but it was evident to me that she felt motivated to examine a shift that had been happening inside of her.

She continued, "It seems like wherever I go, I'm always the person who tries harder and makes the effort with people who seem unattainable to me. But then when people actually *do* care? I find someone else to go after. It's like I get disinterested or something."

Sharee paused for a moment and sighed.

"There are *so* many people who've conveyed that they *see me* or they *care* about my work and opinions. And I hate to say it—but I never care as much about *their* attention. It's like I get bored if someone is kind to me. Instead, it seems I'm most drawn to the people who pay the least attention to me; the ones who make it evident that they don't have time for me or they couldn't care less about my well-being.

"I've realized this for a while now . . . but something in me snapped recently. I am absolutely exhausted from this cycle of going after people and experiences that end up hurting me."

As Sharee and I continued our work together, one thing became evident— her sense that she mattered only if she could impress the least interested person in the room meant that unless and until that happened, she didn't feel she could rest or take care of herself. This, in turn, led to a sense of malnourishment around safety and goodness.

Gently, we began to uncover the way her desire to impress unattainable people was intertwined with her desire to please her highly critical and emotionally unavailable father. As a child, she would daydream about how to make her dad proud of her; and every once in a great while she succeeded. But it was so fleeting; it never satisfied her deep longing to be valued and seen— and it also meant she rarely felt like she could take in glimmers of goodness when they came her way.

"Sharee, what comes up for you when I invite you to notice the progress you're making?" I asked one afternoon. Sharee had just mentioned that instead of dropping everything when her ex-boyfriend texted her out of the blue to join him for a concert, she remembered how often she was left anxious and angry when he would suddenly ghost her for weeks. Sharee then stuck with her plans to hang out with her group of core friends at a barbecue—and this was a *huge* victory for her.

Sharee considered my question and then took a sip of her tea. "It's like as soon as I try to connect with the satisfaction and happiness I feel—because I *know* what would've happened if I started that whole cycle of being available at the drop of a hat—I start to feel shame," she replied.

I asked Sharee if she noticed where she felt shame in her body. Then I asked, "If that sensation could speak, what would it say?"

Sharee's answer didn't come quickly, but as I stayed attuned to her, she replied, "The sensation would say: Who do you think you are? You don't deserve to feel good; you're never going to find someone who really appreciates you."

As Sharee spoke, tears began to stream down her face. "Ugh, I hate that this is what I feel, Aundi—but it's true. It's what I've believed all my life."

The pain didn't magically go away that day, but Sharee told me it felt supportive to have me see and hear her. Over time, using both an attachment lens as well as compassionate resourcing, she came to honor the wound behind that shame: the need to be loved and attuned to by her dad. Consequently, the part of Sharee who thought that she wasn't worthy of goodness began to soften. Slowly she began to accept the nourishment of care she had been deprived of for so long.

As we've discussed in *Strong like Water*, goodness and safety aren't extras. They are not superfluous. In many ways, they're the main event; they give us the ability to move through hard things and be fully human.

As we continued in therapy, Sharee and I focused on helping her build a multitude of compassionate resources to tap into. Initially, this involved establishing practices like grounding, containment, and mindfulness to support Sharee when she would move toward situational strength. But in addition to that, I taught Sharee some of the practices I introduce in *Strong like Water*, such as how to harness "glimmers" (page 137), use the ART tool (page 127), build relational with-ness (page 105), and utilize attachment scripts to help communicate with the people in her life who were showing up for her (page 94).

As Sharee grew, she found that instead of needing a fleeting moment of attention from someone who didn't really care about her, she could honor her pain, reparent herself, and provide the care she needed so she could choose to build relationships with people who valued her too.

BODY-CENTERED EXERCISE

Pages 147–151 of *Strong like Water* describe various types of compassionate resources that might be available to you. In fact, anything your body experiences as safe (or put another way, anything that activates your vagus nerve, thereby communicating safety to your body) can be a resource.

Below I've listed some additional ideas for compassionate resources to gather and harness in your journey. (For a reminder on how to anchor these resources, you may wish to check out page 146 of *Strong like Water*.)

RELATIONAL RESOURCES

In addition to the prompts from the book, feel free to use this space to name other experiences that you have had or are having that feel connected to this type of resource. Examples might include feeling heard or seen; being validated; experiencing a sense of settledness with someone; being with a child, friend, or loved one in a way that feels good; or experiencing fun or lightness with someone in a way that has felt pleasant to you. (As a reminder, if you have few of these experiences, this is not a cause for shame. Instead, I invite you to begin to hunt for goodness as you continue to build your compassionate resources.)

PHYSICAL RESOURCES

In addition to the prompts from the book, I invite you to use this space to name other physical resources that feel good or supportive to you. Perhaps you might think about places you'd like to travel to—and what you notice in your body as you consider those aspirations. Other examples might include new experiences in nature. For instance, I now live in Michigan and am deeply enjoying the experience of different seasons and how they can change a place—the fiery-looking trees in autumn, the glisten of new snow in winter, the iconic spring tulips, and finally, the intensity of summer sunsets over Lake Michigan. My dear friend and fellow writer Kayla Craig writes about the value and beauty of seasons in her book *Every Season Sacred*: "Seasons help us understand our physical and emotional growth, and they guide us into a deeper understanding of our relationship with God."[1] You might consider that for yourself. Is there a resource from each season that feels good or supportive to you?

BOUNDARY RESOURCES

Learning how to set boundaries can be an important part of compassionate resourcing because it helps us build the safety needed to be able to attune to ourselves and ultimately to others as well. Take a moment and consider the way your own body provides an example of the limits we all have; each person has a literal physical place where their body ends and another person begins. No person can do everything or be everything, and this is as it should be. We are finite creatures.

If it feels like a resource, notice the wisdom embedded in your design. Consider this the next time you feel like you are required to do everything, be everything, and say yes to everyone. You may also consider noting anything else that feels supportive (e.g., quotes, affirmations, experiences) as you continue to engage boundaries as a resource.

SPIRITUAL RESOURCES

As I noted in *Strong like Water* and want to reiterate here, I am deeply mindful that faith can be an extraordinary resource—*but* for many people, it has not always been so. The reasons for this can be complex. Perhaps faith or spirituality was weaponized against you or used to harm you. In my own story, I have experienced the tension of wanting to believe God was good to me yet not being able to internalize that into my experience, primarily because of trauma done in the name of Jesus. It has taken deep work, lots of support, and the continued steady kindness of God to relearn something that has not always felt safe. With that said, I want you to know that wherever you are on your journey, you are welcome here. I believe God's heart is deeply kind toward you in your pain.

OBJECTS AS RESOURCES

We know that our bodies are constantly looking for cues of safety, and that even includes the items around us. Are any objects particularly supportive or inspiring to you right now (e.g., a soft blanket, work of art, sweatshirt, candle, essential oils, or books)?

EXPERIENCES AS RESOURCES

Finally, remember that our nervous system is constantly being shaped by our experiences. In the same way that we can be shaped by harm or pain, we can also learn to intentionally engage with reparative work that can move us along the flow of strength. Take a moment to consider any experiences that have felt reparative or supportive for you, such as completing something challenging, doing something playful, apologizing and/or receiving an apology, going on an adventure, trying something new, or attending a concert.

What compassionate resources can you tap into?

RELATIONAL RESOURCES

PHYSICAL RESOURCES

BOUNDARY RESOURCES

SPIRITUAL RESOURCES

OBJECTS AS RESOURCES

EXPERIENCES AS RESOURCES

INVITATION TO REFLECT AND DISCUSS

1. A key concept introduced in chapter 5 of *Strong like Water* is that of internalized safety, which is when we begin to embody the care we've been given so that it affects our internal templates. Ideally, this happened when we experienced "good enough parenting" from our caregivers. When we integrate this skill, the support, resources, or goodness we received doesn't exist only outside of us; it's as though our bodies are better able to hold on to them. How do you think that developing internalized safety relates to moving along the flow of strength?

2. For many people, learning to internalize safety takes time and may even be a delayed process—often because they experienced inconsistent caregiving or systems that taught them it's not safe to hold on to goodness. Has this been true in your own life? How has it affected your daily life, including your ability to have self-compassion?

3. How do you think the concept of internalized safety relates to inner trust? What do you think it means to participate with God as we learn to trust ourselves?

4. On pages 114–115 of *Strong like Water*, I list a few ways that you might recognize moments of transitional strength in your life. Which, if any, resonate with you? If possible, reflect on the context of the situation and how you were able to access that transitional resilience.

5. Why do you think that learning to honor our attachment style and wounds matters to our strong-like-water work?

6. On page 137 of *Strong like Water*, I discuss the concept of "glimmers," a term coined by therapist Deb Dana. If it feels possible to you, take a moment and reflect on any glimmers you may have experienced today. If it feels like a resource, practice taking a moment longer than normal to savor that which you've experienced as a "micro moment" of goodness, safety, connection, or regulation.

7. The psalmist writes, "I remain confident of this: I will see the goodness of the LORD in the land of the living" (Psalm 27:13). What does that verse bring up for you? What do you think is meant by "the goodness of the LORD"?

8. Is there something you feel like you need to say to God but haven't felt able to? If it feels like a resource to you, please feel free to write about that here:

9. I often refer to reminders of God's faithfulness in my life as Ebenezers, or what the Israelites called "stones of help" (see 1 Samuel 7:7-12). In many ways these "stones" have become resources to me when I am feeling alone, discouraged, or isolated. This helps me to remember how God has shown up for me, even in small ways. If it seems beneficial to you, name any "stones of help" in your own life below.

10. Are there any other spiritual practices that you are experiencing as particularly nourishing in the season you are in?

11. What do you think the difference is between true goodness and something such as toxic positivity or spiritual bypassing (see the chart on pages 26–27 of *Strong like Water*)? Why do you think knowing this difference matters?

12. On page 135 of *Strong like Water*, compassionate resources are referred to as the Bubble Wrap that keeps experiences from feeling harmful. If you can, describe a time when you experienced this.

INVITATION TO JOURNAL

We are often taught to *think* our feelings rather than *feel* our feelings; for example, talking about how angry/sad we are instead of physically yelling/crying. When we solely intellectualize our experiences, however, we remain disembodied and ultimately unable to move along the flow of strength through our compassionate resourcing. Overintellectualizing our experience keeps us disconnected from that which could actually help us shift toward healing.

This journaling prompt encourages you to explore resources from a different perspective—an embodied one. I invite you to use the two columns on the next page. Under Life-Giving, you might list people, experiences, or things that feel supportive, spark curiosity, feel spacious, or draw you toward them. Under Life-Draining, you might name people, experiences, or things that deplete you in some way. The work here is to practice engaging with experiences that give you micro moments of lightness, hope, opening, goodness, calm, care, or anything else that feels supportive to your body, mind, and/or soul. On the other side, using the sensations of your body, you are trying to discern what feels like a drain on each of them.

Take a moment now to create your own lists. As you do so, I invite you to be as honest as possible about which activity, experience, person, etc., goes on each side. As a gentle reminder, if someone or something is important to you but is on the draining side of the paper, it doesn't mean that it is inherently bad. In fact, there may be beautiful, meaningful elements to the draining side. (However, we are working to practice radical honesty about how our bodies currently respond to these elements.)

One last tip before you begin: When you think about a larger category like work, see if you can break it into smaller elements. So perhaps you will list administrative work on the life-draining side but place connecting with a client on the life-giving side. Another example is parenting. You might name which elements of parenting feel draining while also parsing out which feel life-giving.

LIFE-GIVING   LIFE-DRAINING

Now that you've written your lists, take a moment to notice how it feels when you consider the items on each side.

Next, pick one or two ideas or concepts from the life-giving side. If it feels like a resource, jot down a few ways you might be able to creatively integrate this more often into your life. You could write about a time that this compassionate resource has already been available to you or a way you would like to shift your time and focus to connect more with this resource.

INVITATION TO CREATE

For our creative activity, we are going to put together a collage of hope. I invite you to gather or draw images, words, colors, or anything else that activates glimmers of goodness for you. You might consider flipping through a magazine and cutting out different images that stand out to you, but please don't be limited by that. Feel free to use whatever materials might contribute to the potential resource you're creating. As you are on the hunt, I encourage you to continue to stay connected to your body as you curiously investigate what you'd like to put into your collage, remembering that the embodied element is part of what makes this work different from spiritual bypassing or toxic positivity.

Seek to create something that is less about its objective value to anyone else and more about how it represents a sense of goodness to you. Once you're finished, consider sharing it with someone you feel could help you honor what you've created.

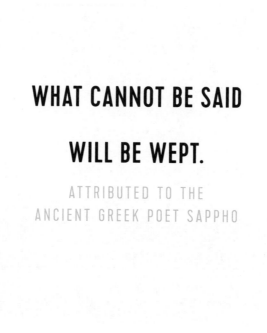

WHAT CANNOT BE SAID

WILL BE WEPT.

ATTRIBUTED TO THE
ANCIENT GREEK POET SAPPHO

EMBRACING THE EBB AND FLOW

A Deeper Dive into Chapters 7 and 8 of *Strong like Water*

WHEN I TRULY BEGAN TO HEAL from years of unaddressed childhood trauma, a curious thing happened: I started to cry at just about every little thing.

I would cry when watching certain commercials. When singing worship songs. When perusing the greeting card aisle. When my husband remembered to say thank you. When he forgot to say thank you. When I received a gift. When I journaled. When I spoke with my mentor. When I spoke with my therapist. When I spoke about my trauma, and even sometimes when I wanted to take a break from talking about my trauma. My tears became a companion in a way I had never experienced before.

Certainly, I had always been a big feeler. But unbeknownst to me, most people didn't perceive me that way. In the midst of coping with a tumultuous and, at times, traumatic home, I had become quite skilled at internalizing and suppressing my feelings—even my terror. Sometimes I'd let emotions out in spurts, or I would channel them into sports or academics—but mostly, I felt the heavy weight of needing to look okay on the outside; I carried the dread in my stomach like a bag of rocks. Most folks in my life had no idea how much I was hurting.

When the tears finally began to fall like floodwaters unleashed from a dam, I was twenty-four, newly graduated with a master's degree in counseling and working to become a licensed professional counselor. But oh my, I had a lot to learn as I aimed to become what Henri Nouwen called a "wounded healer."[1] At the time, much of my focus was on trying to understand the theories and ideas behind psychology, how they integrate with theology, and what it means to walk alongside folks who are suffering. However, what I needed to learn was that the nearness and with-ness of Jesus was deeply accessible to me too. And it always had been—yet because my body had needed to do all she could to survive in my early years, it had been hard to live from that reality.

I look back at that season of ever-present tears as "the great thaw." After being stuck in situational strength for so long, my body needed a way to metabolize the intensity of what she'd experienced. And this, in and of itself, was a compassionate resource to my body—the ability to feel what needed to be felt.

As we continue our strong-like-water work, I invite you to explore ways you, too, can deepen and widen your capacity to experience your emotions.

BODY-CENTERED EXERCISE

Our God-given bodies matter. They allow us to show up in the world; to experience connection, goodness, and beauty. And they are also uniquely equipped to help us metabolize emotions and complete the stress cycle, discharging any energy created in a threatening or intense situation. However, for so many reasons, we often live in deeply disembodied ways; perhaps at some point it didn't feel safe or actually wasn't safe to be fully present mind, body, and spirit.

STRONG-LIKE-WATER LANGUAGE

As we begin to find a new way to be in the world, we often need new language to help honor our experiences. Below I've created a strong-like-water affirmation list that may be a resource to you as you begin to find words that match what you are learning—or even the glimmers of hope and courage that are emerging. If it feels like a support to you, consider bringing in these affirmations as you find them helpful, such as when you are working to reparent a part of yourself, needing to convey self-compassion instead of shame, or working to soothe yourself when you are feeling dysregulated. Feel free to take only what you need from the list (and add to it as you learn more about what your unique system needs to hear).

- I can be soft and fierce.

- I can find people who help my body exhale.

- I can feel my emotions at the pace I am able.

- What once served me may no longer serve me.

- Surviving is good, but I am allowed to do more than exist.

- Discomfort is okay; harm is not.

- I can honor the pace of my body.

- Compassion will lead the way.

To engage in a deeper embodiment and move toward integrated strength, I invite you to try a practice that will help you "show over tell" your body that you are safe and can be present within it, as well as ultimately move the energy of stressful experiences through your body.

First, ensure that you are in a grounded place. (See page 95 if you'd like a refresher on this practice.) Now I invite you to consider a situation—not your biggest trauma, but perhaps a mild irritation. Next, as you are able, do a body scan as you reflect on this experience.

For example, perhaps you are thinking of being stuck in traffic, going to the grocery store when it's busy, or having to scroll by a comment on social media that might automatically make you brace. As you bring this frustrating event into your mind's eye, what are you noticing?

Next, as you are able, take a moment to let yourself embody the tension that you're feeling. For example, take a moment and clench your fists, bring up your shoulders, tighten your chest—do with your body everything that the annoying experience makes you want to do.

Then, mindfully, and with as much compassion as you're able, I invite you to intentionally

feel your feet on the ground
unclench your hands and fingers
lower your shoulders
loosen your jaw
lift your chin
soften your gaze
slow your breathing and lengthen your exhale

Once you've done some or all of these, take a moment and tune in to what you're noticing. Have these actions shifted how you relate to what you've brought up in your mind's eye? If they have and this practice feels like a resource to you, I invite you to notice and savor the spaciousness you may be feeling.

If any tension and/or unsettledness remains, can you get curious about what else needs to happen for your body to move through what you're experiencing? In chapter 8 of *Strong like Water*, I talk about Luisa and the additional support she needed to complete the cycle in her own body. Similarly, you may need to incorporate some additional practices to cycle through your own experience.

Check in with your body to see if it might be helpful to

shake your hands, feet, or any other part of your body

roll your head or neck

sway or rock

yawn or hum

cross your arms and press lightly on your arms or shoulders
    (sometimes known as a butterfly hug)

stomp your feet

lengthen your exhale

run in place

press your hands against a wall

turn on loud, energetic music and dance

turn on soft, slow music and dance

You could also choose several of these to practice and experiment with at the same time as you complete the cycle in your own body.

After going through some of these movements, notice what you are experiencing. Has anything changed in your body? While each person's experience is unique, you may notice a sense of heat or tingling; or perhaps an internal shifting, as though you are coming to the end of a wave of emotion. This might be evidenced through tears, deep sighs, or even a sense of settledness. These may be cues to your system that you are metabolizing and completing your own stress cycle. As always, I invite you to stay curious and compassionate as you continue to attune to your own body.

INVITATION TO REFLECT AND DISCUSS

1. Do you typically view the concept of flexibility as a source of strength?
   Why or why not?

2. Is there anywhere in your life that you experience what Dr. Arielle Schwartz refers
   to as safe mobilization (see *Strong like Water*, page 170)? In other words, are you
   able to move your body in a way that feels safe and supportive to you (e.g., through
   play, sports, or other activities)? If so, describe. If not, consider what type of activity
   might feel like a resource to you, and how you might find space to engage in it at
   some point.

3. Similarly, consider whether you have any experience with safe *immobilization* (see *Strong like Water*, pages 170–171). Are you able to settle your body in a way that feels safe and supportive to you (e.g., through rest, sleep, stillness, meditation, or prayer)? If so, describe. If not, consider what type of activity might feel like a resource to you, and how you might find space to engage in it at some point.

4. Scholars sometimes disagree on the exact number, but note that roughly 30 to 65 percent of the Psalms center on themes of lament, sadness, and pain.[2] Do you find that this emphasis on lament is reflected in the way the church discusses and/ or talks about grief or pain? Are there any shifts you would like to see churches make in this area? How might you contribute to that change?

5. If you feel comfortable doing so, share any compassionate resource you find useful as you seek to feel your emotions (e.g., remembering a specific Bible verse; journaling; talking; breathing; listening to music; or engaging in titration, pendulation, prayer, or movement).

6. What barriers, if any, do you experience when you aim to be emotionally flexible?

7. Repatterning is a way to both "process past pain or trauma" and "lay new neural pathways to support us in a different physical response" (*Strong like Water*, page 195). What areas of wounding or growth would you like to continue to repattern in your own life? What compassionate resources might you need to do so?

8. Are there any particular elements of Jesus' life that feel like a resource when you consider the concept of nervous system flexibility? For example, you may reflect on the way Jesus took time away from the crowds after busy periods in ministry (Mark 1:35; Luke 6:12), became angry at injustice (Matthew 21:12-13; Mark 10:14-16), wept with grief (John 11:35), engaged with celebration (John 2:1-11), and even expressed anxiety and panic to His Father in the garden of Gethsemane (Matthew 26:38-39; Luke 22:41-44). As you consider these different expressions of Jesus' humanity, do they help you in any way to have compassion toward your own?

PROMPTS TO CONSIDER AS YOU
THINK ABOUT REPATTERNING

1. Briefly scan your body from head to toe.

2. As you do, take note of what you are experiencing right now. If any part of your body feels "tight or contracted," as Dr. Schwartz describes it, you may benefit from answering the following prompts:

   · Where in your body are you experiencing these sensations (e.g., tension in your neck, trembling hands, pounding heart, heaviness in your chest)? If you notice any of these reactions—or something altogether different—see if you can utilize curiosity to try a different way to move your body:

     For tightness in your shoulders, explore movement or touch.
     For a lump in the throat, explore making different sounds.
     For trembling hands, notice what it feels like to tighten and then loosen them.
     For a pounding heart, place your hand on your heart and notice what it feels like to be supported.
     For heaviness in your chest, give yourself a bear hug and notice what that support feels like.

Each of the prompts above is merely a suggestion and an invitation to bring curiosity to the way your body may need to move in order to move through the cycle of whatever you're feeling. Please add to or tweak these suggestions based on what you are experiencing.[3]

INVITATION TO JOURNAL

Though it seems counterintuitive, the ability to truly grieve is a core part of health because it facilitates the mechanisms that allow our bodies to metabolize pain. Yet in Western culture, grief can be seen either as a type of flaw—something to be put away or checked off a list—or as something you need to commodify, to put on display.

But in many ways, neither of these approaches allows us to truly grieve because neither is based on internal listening; instead, they are rooted in an outward orientation. Total avoidance and/or performance of grief may be forms of situational strength that keep us from actually attending to the pain that needs tending. In her book *A Hole in the World*, Amanda Held Opelt, whose sister, Rachel Held Evans, died unexpectedly at thirty-seven, writes, "There is no life hack for grief. . . . The ability to grieve deeply is a survival skill, one we've come close to losing as a society."[4]

I tend to agree with Amanda. In order to grieve, our bodies need tethers to a certain amount of safety to connect with our pain in a way that feels accessible. This may be why I find it so beautiful to discuss grief through the lens of lament and being held by God since these truths communicate to our bodies that it's safe to grieve.

In this section, I invite you to first take a moment to ensure you are grounded. Then, notice what you sense in your body when I mention grief. As you do so, consider this question for journaling: Has any experience of grief in your life shaped you? How so?

Alternately, is there an experience or are there experiences that you've needed to grieve but haven't been able to?

What might it look like for you to use strong-like-water principles to compassionately tend that pain?

INVITATION TO CREATE

One way to support your body as you learn to complete cycles of stress is to find ways to externalize the experience—using art, for example, as a compassionate resource.[5] Mindfully attending to what is being experienced in your body allows you to move through an experience, moment, or sensation.

For this activity, you will need a blank piece of paper and a drawing utensil (pencil, marker, paintbrush). Before you begin, I encourage you to ensure you are in a grounded place and experiencing at least a tether of safety in the present.

Next, you may consider either closing your eyes or softening your gaze. Take thirty seconds to a minute to simply notice your breath as you inhale through your nose and exhale through your mouth. Now take your drawing utensil and begin at one side of the paper. As you inhale, show it on your paper by creating an upward curve that matches your breath. As you begin to exhale, turn your curve downward. Spend a few minutes drawing upward and downward curves as you inhale and exhale. Your finished paper may look something like this (with your own unique curves, of course):

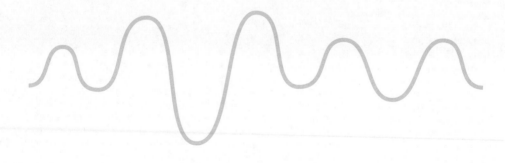

I THINK THE SAME THOUGHTS

AGAIN AND AGAIN:

LIFE IS SO BEAUTIFUL.

LIFE IS SO HARD.

KATE BOWLER

IN SERVICE OF WHOLENESS

A Deeper Dive into Chapters 9 and 10 of *Strong like Water*

EVERY ONCE IN A WHILE IN MY WORK as a therapist, speaker, and author, I hear from folks who've interacted with my writing or with whom I've done therapy in the past. And because our journeys never function like checklists where things neatly fall into place, they aren't necessarily contacting me to tell me that everything is magically perfect (though it is pretty cool to bear witness to some of the growth that happens). But here's the sort of thing I do often have the privilege of hearing:

> Thank you for teaching me how to listen to my body. Thank you for helping me remember that no matter what happens or where I go, God's posture toward me is deeply kind. Thank you for showing me that I have access to the tools, resources, and even relationships I need to face hard things. I am learning that I can heal. I am learning to come home to myself and be open to the possibilities of restoration.

Reader, I share this with you because in so many ways the work of learning to be strong like water has a profound overlap with the concept of integration and wholeness. From a biblical perspective, wholeness might be thought of as shalom, which Lisa Sharon Harper discusses this way:

> Shalom is what the Kingdom of God smells like. It's what the Kingdom looks like and what Jesus requires of the Kingdom's citizens. It's when everyone has enough. It's when families are healed. It's when shame is renounced and inner freedom is laid hold of. It's when human dignity, bestowed by the image of God in all humanity, is cultivated, protected, and served in families, faith communities, and schools and through public policy. Shalom is when the capacity to lead is recognized in every human being and when nations join together to protect the environment.[1]

I'm moved and inspired by this perspective on shalom, and I believe that through this work, we learn to participate in the greater vision of flourishing available to us—both for our neighbors and for ourselves.

While writing this guided journey, I have been reflecting on this truth. Growing up, I learned to be extremely careful in an effort to avoid triggering my father's explosive anger and abuse. But now, as the trauma that fueled that situational strength has begun to heal, I can see that this need to be careful has transformed into something much more life-giving: being a person who is care-full; that is, full of care. This ability and desire to notice and attend to people's pain compassionately is an outgrowth of the high sensitivity I had to develop toward others' internal states in order to survive. Through experiences of safety, love, compassion, and the grace of God, I have been able to metabolize the hypervigilance and fawning I initially developed in chronic trauma. Care I once offered mostly to maintain some semblance of protection can now be given from a place of true choice. Ultimately my situational strength has been replaced with a deep integrated strength, enabling me to profoundly care for others, even as I care for myself.

As we move along the flow of strength, attend to the wounds present in our stories, come home to the people God created us to be, and continue living into the fullness of our God-given selves, we deepen our compassion for others and ourselves. We find again and again: Healing begets healing. Life begets life.

We remember that when we operate out of situational strength, it doesn't mean we are less valuable or less worthy of care. We do, however, move forward in the already-but-not-yet of wholeness because God's desire and hope for us is always richer, kinder, and more expansive than we may even be able to imagine for ourselves. In so many ways, this is the currency we work in: wholeness.

My deep hope is that you have begun to ask yourself questions like *Will this move me toward integration? Does this act in service of wholeness? Does this action, behavior, or thought support my flourishing or the flourishing of another? (And if it doesn't, what kind of compassionate resource might that part of myself need?)*

This is where the profound goodness seems to seep through: Those things that may have once been *only* in service of survival can often be transformed so that they can now contribute to wholeness. Those things that were meant for harm, somehow, by the mercy of God become part of the tapestry of our strength.

May it be so.

BODY-CENTERED EXERCISE

Pain, trauma, and loss can steal so much from us. It's necessary and worthwhile for us to honor this reality. I will always advocate for honoring our pain because we never heal by pretending or bypassing. As we move toward integrated strength, a phenomenal thing begins—sometimes slowly, other times all at once. We begin to believe that new life is possible.

We, like Mary Magdalene, the first person to lay eyes on the resurrected Jesus, begin to recognize that even after what feels like the final blow— resurrection *is* possible.[2] Somehow, beauty *can* come from ashes. Hope *can* be found even amid despair. Shoots of life somehow burst through even the most barren of landscapes, almost inexplicably creating fields of new blooms. It's important to remember that this doesn't mean we need to be grateful for abuse or trauma, but perhaps it can be a balm to remind us that God is in the business of birthing life from death. Again and again, I come back to this great mystery, and I am moved by it even now.

What does that mean for us in our strong-like-water work, dear reader? It can mean a multitude of things. This is why I say that we need the imagination of artists, poets, prophets, writers, musicians, and all those who have the capacity to view life with a more expansive viewpoint (see *Strong like Water*, pages 229–230). As we partner with God in reimagining our way forward, I invite you to engage the following body-centered practice:

Beginning from a grounded place, situate yourself comfortably, either sitting or standing, and ask yourself these questions, following the prompts as you're able:

- **If you could fully internalize the reality that you are beloved by God, how might that affect your body in this very moment?** Take a moment now, slowing your breath as you feel able, bringing in a compassionate curiosity, and asking yourself, *How might this affect my body?* while doing a body scan.

- **Next, attune to how this question about belovedness is landing for you.** If it feels supportive, explore how you might want to respond to this question. For example, do you sit up straighter? Do your shoulders come up? Or drop down? Do you place a hand on your heart? Does your breathing slow down? Does any internal tension seem to soften? Do you give yourself a gentle hug? (These are only ideas to try if they feel helpful. Ultimately, please stay curious about what feels most authentic to *you* as you reimagine how you experience a sense of yourself as God's beloved.)

As always, if for any reason this practice feels overwhelming or flooding to you, please remember you can discontinue it at any time. Second, if you are not able to connect with the original invitation around belovedness, please be gentle with yourself. Perhaps try this instead: Imagine someone else you believe God sees as beloved. As you see them in your mind's eye, go through a similar practice as you consider how that knowledge affects *your* body. Now, see if it might be possible for you to imagine yourself alongside this person, also remaining curious about your own belovedness.

You can stay with either of these practices as long as it seems helpful to you. Please feel free to adapt this practice in ways that it might continue to support you, such as by asking:

What would I say if I could internalize that I am God's beloved?
What would I write?
How would I act?
How would I live?

INVITATION TO REFLECT AND DISCUSS

1. In the opening section I discuss how my tendency to be "careful" has, through experiences of repair, been transformed into an ability to be full of care for others. Have you ever had an experience where something that was once a survival strategy seemed to transform into something that now works for your good? If so, explain.

2. What do you think is meant by the phrase "in service of wholeness"?

3. How does the concept of wholeness seem to intersect with the biblical concept
of shalom?

4. What or who comes to mind when you consider the phrase "courageous hope" (*Strong
like Water*, page 229)? How might people understand the verse "be strong and
courageous" (Joshua 1:9) differently when viewed through the lens of being strong like
water rather than relying on traditional strength (e.g., white-knuckling through pain)?

5. Sometimes our growth means we will "appear different from what others desire for and of us" (*Strong like Water*, page 221). How have you experienced that to be true in your own life? How does Jesus model disappointing people in a healthy way at times?

SHOOTS OF LIFE SOMEHOW

BURST THROUGH EVEN THE

MOST BARREN OF LANDSCAPES,

ALMOST INEXPLICABLY CREATING

FIELDS OF NEW BLOOMS.

INVITATION TO JOURNAL

In chapter 9 of *Strong like Water*, reflecting on my profound experience on the Oregon coast, I share, "I realized something new about the work of becoming strong like water: My truest, most profound strength will never be found in denying the reality of my personhood or my story. Instead, the deepest strength has always, always been about welcoming them home" (page 207).

When you read that quote, I invite you to notice what comes up in your own body. Does it feel easy to accept or perhaps a little difficult to agree with? Take a moment and simply answer this question for yourself. If you, too, have at times experienced moments of integration and/or integrated strength, you may also take a moment to reflect on that. Feel free to jot down any words or phrases that come up for you as you do.

Next, as you feel able, consider what it might be like for you to welcome parts of yourself or your story that have felt exiled. Please be aware, as always, that the more complicated your trauma, the more complex the healing will be. There is no shame in this; in fact, it makes a lot of sense. If you have a history of unresolved trauma, you may find that you feel disconnected from many aspects of yourself and your story. As always, we want to honor our pace in the welcoming home.

If it feels accessible to you, take a moment and write about what comes up for you when I extend this invitation. If it feels like a resource to practice a gentle faith integration, you may consider the posture and compassion of the father in the story of the Prodigal Son (Luke 15:11-32). What do you notice in your body when you consider the tenderness of the father? What would it be like for you to receive this type of care? You may or may not resonate with this young man, but remember that "while he was still a long way off, his father saw him and was filled with compassion for him; he ran to his son, threw his arms around him and kissed him" (Luke 15:20). This is God's exact posture toward you, and you are invited to participate with God in welcoming home any part of yourself that has not felt safe enough to do so.

For the final part of this journal practice, I want to invite you to write a letter to any part of yourself from which you have felt disconnected.

For example, in *Strong like Water* I share the fierce part of myself who developed in my childhood, especially while playing basketball. In my early adulthood, I felt ambivalent toward this part. From a trauma lens, this fierce me had been (rightly) carrying deep anger about the way I had been treated in my childhood. But because this part of me was so young, it didn't know what to *do* with that anger—it didn't have enough compassionate resourcing to metabolize the emotion. Therefore, as an adult, it sometimes felt overwhelming to come into contact with this part of myself; in my own work of integration, I had to build trust with this younger part so it could begin to recognize that I was there to help compassionately resource it the way it desperately needed.

AFFIRMATIONS FOR COMING HOME TO YOURSELF

I am listening.

You are not alone.

It makes sense to feel _____.

It's okay to feel what you feel.

We will work together to figure this out.

I'm not going anywhere.

Your pace is valid.

Your grief is real.

I will stay as close as it feels helpful.

God is with us.

We are beloved.

INVITATION TO CREATE

Author Susan Cain writes, "Whatever pain you can't get rid of, make it your creative offering."[3] In her book *Bittersweet*, she shows the ways it's possible for pain to ultimately be transformed into beauty, art, and goodness; and in many ways, I find this to be a model for the spiritual life. Somehow the soil of our grief and heartache can become the fertile ground for new life to be born. There is a sacred mystery that happens as we bring our wounds to the Good Shepherd. This is the God who tends us in ways beyond our human imagination and, what's more, empowers us to participate in stewarding compassionate resources to ourselves too. Our good, kind God knows how we are made; knows that when pain or trauma occurs, it's rarely a matter of simply getting over it. Instead, we must have various avenues that allow our bodies to move through the pain—and sometimes, one of those avenues is creativity. God knows how our bodies, minds, and spirits need ways to transmute that which we have been carrying, and often this is deeply intertwined with the work that happens as we move toward integration.

For our final creative resource, I invite you to a two-part creative practice that I hope will help support you as you continue to embody healing. Begin by gathering art materials—paper and watercolors, oil paints, crayons, markers, or chalk.

Then take a moment to ground yourself. Next, consider an area of your life in which you hope to see healing or growth. Perhaps you still feel a sense of pain or disturbance connected to it, and that's okay. In your mind's eye, see if you can offer compassion to the part of yourself or your story that feels "unfinished."

As you remain connected to what you're noticing, see if you can create a drawn or painted image that helps you externalize what you're feeling internally. As you do this, notice the colors you tend toward; the intensity and variation of the hues. Notice the designs you want to make. Notice how much space you want to take up. Notice what it feels like to transfer your feelings onto paper. I encourage you to remember that your creation can be as subjective as you would like; the only person it needs to be symbolic or meaningful for is you.

At a later time (it could be as short as thirty minutes or much longer), come back to the artwork you created. Now if you feel comfortable doing so, I invite you to reimagine what you've created. (At first, this may seem strange, but I encourage you to think of this as an experiment.) Here are some ideas to spur you on in your own process:

- Rip up the art you created into little pieces and repaste it to make new art.
- Cut it into strips and make an entirely new picture.
- Write words on the original picture that parts of you need to hear.
- Add layer or texture over what you've already created to bring out something new.

Once you've done this, notice what's it's like for that which represented pain to be transformed into something entirely different. If it feels helpful for you, find a person or a group of people with whom you can share your insights.

BENEDICTION

DEAR ONE, AS ALWAYS, it is a privilege to walk alongside you in the work of healing. Thank you for joining me in these pages. I pray they have somehow served you, and perhaps have even created new sparks of hope and imagination as to what may be possible in this beautiful, difficult, glorious life we've each been offered.

As you continue in your strong-like-water journey, may you have eyes to see that though the reality of pain is great, so, too, is the reality of goodness. May you come to know that the spaciousness of healing is available not just to others but also to you. As you engage with this deep work, may you find that the flow of strength has already been embedded in you by a Good Creator. You need only to enter this grace that is already available to you.

In the ebb and flow of your growth, may you relentlessly return to the "ground of your being"—the God who loves you, forms you, and calls you beloved. May our kind God, the great co-regulator and author of compassion and goodness, be nearer to you than you could have imagined as you learn to move with the Spirit in your healing work.

Aundi Kolber
June 2023

YOU NEED ONLY TO

ENTER THIS GRACE

THAT IS ALREADY

AVAILABLE TO YOU.

GUIDANCE FOR GROUP LEADERS

LEARNING AND GROWING IN COMMUNITY are essential parts of what it means to be human. Yet as the old adage goes, we are both "harmed in relationship and healed in relationship." Because this is true, my hope is that folks who participate in a discussion group feel empowered to have both a voice and a choice in the work of becoming strong like water, and that their involvement inspires self-attunement throughout. Practicing and encouraging this compassionate posture also supports us as we seek to love our neighbors as ourselves.

With this in mind, I've laid out a few recommendations for basic guidelines on how to facilitate a discussion group that seeks to integrate trauma-informed principles. As always, the group itself and the individuals within it can choose what works best. Seek to honor choice, autonomy, and self-attunement in the group by

- encouraging group members to answer or not answer questions, depending on what feels helpful to them;
- encouraging group members to be aware of their own windows of tolerance and utilize skills to ground themselves if they become overwhelmed;
- encouraging members to take breaks (e.g., use the restroom, get a drink of water, have a snack) as needed throughout the group time in order to attune to themselves;

- encouraging group members to honor each other's limits when someone chooses not to participate in part of a discussion;
- encouraging group members to seek professional care if or when the content or process of the group surpasses what the group can offer in terms of support; and
- encouraging group members to seek professional trauma-informed care if or when they find they'd like to continue to process themes that have come up in the group.

GROUNDING RESOURCE

One resource I frequently teach to folks I work with and utilize in my own life is grounding.[1] Clinical psychologist and trauma expert Dr. Arielle Schwartz notes that grounding "refers to our ability to experience ourselves as embodied . . . to sense [our] body, feel [our] feet on the earth, and as a result calm [our] nervous system."[2] We engage our five senses to the extent that we are able to bring our body and awareness into the present. We do this because, God willing, the present moment is safe—or at least safer than the moments we are recalling when we feel flooded or overwhelmed.

Though there are many ways to practice grounding, one simple way is to engage the language of *noticing* as you use your different senses. You can do this practice anywhere, although if possible, it's especially helpful to get outside.

To begin, use this language with yourself as you actively seek out:

a. "I'm noticing [something I can see] _____".
b. "I'm noticing [something I can touch] _____".
c. "I'm noticing [something I can hear] _____".
d. "I'm noticing [something I can smell] _____".
e. "I'm noticing [something I can taste] _____".

I invite you to continue to use this practice until you begin to feel more regulated or for as long as it feels helpful. As always, if at any point this resource starts to make you feel further triggered or flooded, you can discontinue it.

CONTAINMENT RESOURCE

There are times it's not only appropriate but also *necessary* to create some internal space between ourselves and that which feels too disturbing or overwhelming to connect with. When this is the case, we can create a psychological "container" to help us create this space.[1] We don't use containment to suppress pain but instead to mindfully access it in a way that restores choice—we get to decide how we engage with it. Often trauma survivors have had little power in moments or experiences that were disturbing, so the hope is that practices like these can be a part of the repair.

1. In your mind's eye, consider an object or space that feels like it might be able to "hold" the disturbance you're experiencing. Please know you can be as creative with this as feels helpful. For example, I've had clients picture placing their overwhelm in a spaceship and launching it into the sky, putting their pain in a huge safe, or even picturing God's hands holding the disturbance for them.

2. After you have your "container" in your mind's eye, consider what feels disturbing or overwhelming as you scan your body from head to toe. (If this is your first time doing this practice, I recommend choosing something mildly disturbing/irritating to practice with.) As you consider your disturbance, picture a laser starting at your head and going all the way to your toes to locate where in your body you feel it. After you've located it in your body, take a moment to see if you can place this disturbance in your container. Know that you can take as long as you need to fully place the disturbance all the way into the container.

3. As you do this, your body is going to give you the best information as to whether your container is "strong" enough. If you begin to feel some relief after placing your disturbance in the container, this is a sign that the container is sufficient. However, if you don't experience relief, you may consider placing your original container into an additional container(s) to create more layers between you and the disturbance. For example, you could take a bank vault you imagined and then place that entire vault at the bottom of the ocean.

4. Finally, once you experience that sense of space, name your container. Take a moment and notice the space you feel and then create a name that helps convey what you're feeling.

If at any point this practice no longer feels helpful, you may wish to begin with grounding, contain whatever still feels disturbing, and then go back to grounding. As always, I encourage you to reach out to a licensed therapist if you need additional support.

NOTES

INTRODUCTION

1. Tasha Jun (@tashajunb), Instagram, April 1, 2021, https://www.instagram.com/p/CNIIqfvLv1E/.
2. I first used this structure in *The Try Softer Guided Journey* (Tyndale Refresh, 2021) and was pleased to hear from readers that it enabled them to personalize and apply the concepts introduced in the companion book.
3. Daniel J. Siegel, *Mindsight: The New Science of Personal Transformation* (New York: Bantam Books, 2010), 107–108.

SESSION 1: EMBODIED PAIN REQUIRES EMBODIED HEALING

1. Arielle Schwartz, *The Complex PTSD Workbook: A Mind-Body Approach to Regaining Emotional Control and Becoming Whole* (Berkeley, CA: Althea Press, 2016), 85.
2. I originally learned about the importance of a somatic vocabulary at a training that integrates EMDR with somatic psychology in July 2017. This list is one I've compiled as I've worked with clients.
3. Inspired by Thomas Keating's Welcoming Prayer. See *Strong like Water*, pages 57–58.
4. United States Geological Survey, "The Water in You: Water and the Human Body," May 22, 2019, https://www.usgs.gov/special-topics/water-science-school/science/water-you-water-and -human-body.

SESSION 2: TENDING THE ACHE FOR COMPASSIONATE WITH-NESS

1. Dr. Peter Levine discusses this in his book *Waking the Tiger: Healing Trauma* (Berkeley, CA: North Atlantic Books, 1997), 16–18.
2. See Kristin Neff, *Self-Compassion: The Proven Power of Being Kind to Yourself* (New York: William Morrow, 2011).
3. Deb Dana, *The Polyvagal Theory in Therapy: Engaging the Rhythm of Regulation* (New York: W. W. Norton, 2018), xviii.
4. This is a common art therapy practice that helps to externalize what we may know in our bodies but may not yet be consciously aware of.

SESSION 3: THE WISDOM OF GOODNESS

1. Kayla Craig, *Every Season Sacred: Reflections, Prayers, and Invitations to Nourish Your Soul and Nurture Your Family throughout the Year* (Carol Stream, IL: Tyndale Refresh, 2023), 1.

SESSION 4: EMBRACING THE EBB AND FLOW

1. Henri J. M. Nouwen, *The Wounded Healer: Ministry in Contemporary Society* (New York: Image Books, 1972).
2. Scholars differ on how to categorize various psalms, which may be why there is some disagreement on the exact percentage of lament. My data for this range comes from two sources: "Walter Brueggemann: The Prophetic Imagination," *On Being with Krista Tippett* podcast, December 20, 2018, https://onbeing.org/programs/walter-brueggemann-the-prophetic -imagination-dec2018/; Glenn Packiam, "Five Things to Know about Lament," N. T. Wright Online, accessed July 3, 2023, https://www.ntwrightonline.org/five-things-to-know-about -lament/.
3. I first learned about this concept from Dr. Arielle Schwartz, and this practice is an adaption from one she provides at Arielle Schwartz, "Healing PTSD: Mind and Body in Trauma Treatment," Center for Resilient Informed Therapy blog, August 4, 2020, https://drarielleschwartz.com /healing-ptsd-mind-and-body-in-trauma-treatment-dr-arielle-schwartz/#.YfL5AVjMITU.
4. Amanda Held Opelt, *A Hole in the World: Finding Hope in the Rituals of Grief and Healing* (Franklin, TN: Worthy, 2022), 11.
5. This exercise was inspired by Carolyn Mehlomakulu, "Drawing Your Breath: A Mindful Art Exercise," Creativity in Therapy, August 6, 2017, https://creativityintherapy.com/2017/08 /drawing-your-breath-a-mindful-art-exercise/.

SESSION 5: IN SERVICE OF WHOLENESS

1. Lisa Sharon Harper, *The Very Good Gospel: How Everything Wrong Can Be Made Right* (Colorado Springs, CO: WaterBrook, 2016), 14.
2. See John 20 and Mark 16:9.
3. Susan Cain, *Bittersweet: How Sorrow and Longing Make Us Whole* (New York: Crown, 2022), 56.

GROUNDING RESOURCE

1. I was first introduced to this concept by Barb Maiberger at an EMDR (eye movement desensitization and reprocessing) training session in 2014. Barb also describes a version of this practice in her book *Remote Together: A Therapist's Guide to Cultivating a Sustainable Practice* (Boulder, CO: Bodymind Press, 2021), 304.
2. Arielle Schwartz, "Grounding," Center for Resilience Informed Therapy blog, December 12, 2017, https://drarielleschwartz.com/grounding-dr-arielle-schwartz/#.YjzCqBPMLt0.

CONTAINMENT RESOURCE

1. This is a common resource used in trauma work. I was first introduced to this concept by Barb Maiberger at an EMDR training in 2014.

ABOUT THE AUTHOR

AUNDI KOLBER is a licensed professional counselor (LPC), speaker, and author of the groundbreaking book *Try Softer* and its companion, *The Try Softer Guided Journey.* Aundi is the owner of Kolber Counseling, LLC, established in 2009. She has received additional training in her specialization of trauma- and body-centered therapies, including the highly researched and regarded eye movement desensitization and reprocessing (EMDR) therapy.

Aundi is passionate about the integration of faith and psychology, and is a sought-after expert in both faith and secular settings. She regularly speaks at local and national events, and has appeared on *Good Morning America* as well as podcasts such as *The Lazy Genius* with Kendra Adachi, *Typology*, and *The Next Right Thing* with Emily P. Freeman. Aundi reaches an audience numbering in the tens of thousands via email and social media. You can find her at @aundikolber on Instagram and Twitter or on her website at aundikolber.com.

As a survivor of trauma and a lifelong learner, Aundi brings hard-won knowledge around the work of change, the power of redemption, and the beauty of experiencing God *with* us in our pain. After years of longing to be closer to water, she and her family recently relocated from the majestic mountains of Colorado to the stunning lakes of Michigan. She is happily married to her best friend, Brendan, and is the proud mom of Matia and Jude.

A MORE EXPANSIVE WAY OF HEALING AND STRENGTH IS POSSIBLE.

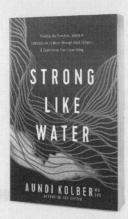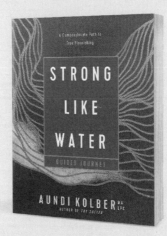

Discover how to internalize connection, love, and safety— empowering you with greater resilience. You were made to be strong like water.

Available wherever books are sold.

CP1956

Also available from Aundi Kolber . . .

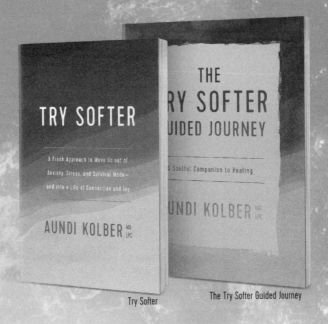

Try Softer

The Try Softer Guided Journey

Trying softer is sacred work. This is what we were made for: a living, breathing, moving, feeling, connected, beautifully incarnational life.

Available wherever books are sold.

CP1822

Tyndale | REFRESH

Think Well. Live Well. Be Well.

Experience the flourishing of your mind, body, and soul with Tyndale Refresh.

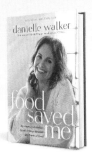

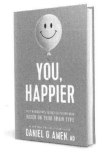

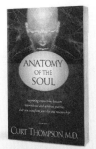

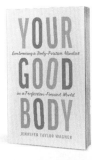

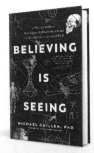

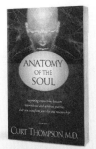

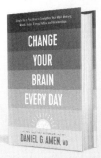

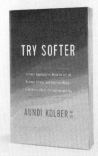

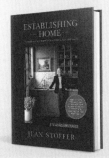

CP1841